THE *Skinny* SLOW COOKER FAST FITNESS

RECIPE & WORKOUT BOOK

D1337438

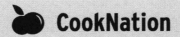

CookNation

THE SKINNY SLOW COOKER/FAST FITNESS RECIPE & WORKOUT BOOK
DELICIOUS CALORIE COUNTED SLOW COOKER MEALS & 15 MINUTE WORKOUTS FOR A LEANER. FITTER YOU

Copyright © Bell & Mackenzie Publishing Limited 2016
All rights reserved. This book or any portion thereof may not be reproduced or used in any manner whatsoever without the express written permission of the publisher.

ISBN 978-1-911219-53-8

• •

DISCLAIMER

Some recipes may contain nuts or traces of nuts. Those suffering from any allergies associated with nuts should avoid any recipes containing nuts or nut based oils.
This information is provided and sold with the knowledge that the publisher and author do not offer any legal or other professional advice.
In the case of a need for any such expertise consult with the appropriate professional.
This book does not contain all information available on the subject, and other sources of recipes are available.

A basic level of fitness is required to perform the workouts in this book. Any health concerns should be discussed with a health professional before embarking on any of the exercises detailed.

This book has not been created to be specific to any individual's requirements. Every effort has been made to make this book as accurate as possible. However, there may be typographical and or content errors. Therefore, this book should serve only as a general guide and not as the ultimate source of subject information.

This book contains information that might be dated and is intended only to educate and entertain.

The author and publisher shall have no liability or responsibility to any person or entity regarding any loss or damage incurred, or alleged to have incurred, directly or indirectly, by the information contained in this book.

CONTENTS

MEALS UNDER 400 CALORIES

MEALS UNDER 500 CALORIES

HIIT PLAN WORKOUTS

OTHER COOKNATION TITLES

INTRODUCTION

Slow cooking & fast fitness make a killer combination

Making time to eat well and exercise regularly isn't always easy. We all lead busy lives and to devote additional time to planning healthy, balanced meals along with going to the gym or exercise classes is often impossible. If you are time poor or perhaps need some motivation, the Skinny Slow Cooker Fast Fitness Recipe & Workout Book is for you. Our easy to prepare yet delicious slow cooker recipes can be prepped in under 15 minutes then left to slowly cook to perfection while you tend to your daily life. Combine this with our step-by-step 15 minute interval training workouts and you have a killer combination to get you on track to a healthier lifestyle without spending hours in the kitchen or the gym.

Our collection of low-calorie recipes will help you make inexpensive, healthy meals for yourself and your family with the minimum of fuss. During the colder months our bodies naturally crave warm, filling and comforting food that can often result in overeating, weight gain and sluggishness. These delicious recipes use simple and inexpensive fresh ingredients; are packed full of flavour and goodness, and show that you can enjoy maximum taste with minimum calories. Each recipe has been tried, tested, and enjoyed time and time again. They are perfect for any calorie controlled diet.

PREPARATION

All of the recipes take no longer than 10-15 minutes to prepare. Browning the meat will make a difference to the taste of your recipe but if you really don't have the time, don't worry, it will still taste good. There are a number of 'shortcut' ingredients throughout this book, but often there is also the option to make these from scratch if you have the time. All meat and vegetables should be cut into even sized pieces. Meat generally cooks faster than vegetables, although root vegetables can take longer, so make sure everything is bite-sized. All meat should be trimmed of visible fat and the skin removed.

NUTRITION

All of the recipes in this collection are balanced low calorie family meals under 500 calories which should keep you feeling full and help you avoid snacking in-between meals. All recipes have serving suggestions; the calories noted are per serving of the recipe ingredients only, so bear that in mind. Most of the recipes serve 4. If you are cooking for one, all the recipes can be frozen for another day.

LOW COST

Slow cooking is ideal for cheaper meat cuts. The 'tougher' cuts used in this collection of recipes are transformed into meat which melts-in-your-mouth and helps to keep the costs down. We've also made sure not to include too many one-off ingredients which are required for a single recipe and never used again. All the herbs and spices listed can be used in multiple recipes throughout the book.

USING YOUR SLOW COOKER: A FEW THINGS

All cooking times are a guide. Make sure you get to know your own slow cooker so that you can adjust timings accordingly. A spray of one cal cooking oil in the cooker before adding ingredients will help with cleaning or you can buy liners. Be confident with your cooking. Feel free to use substitutes to suit your own taste and don't let a missing herb or spice stop you making a meal - you'll almost always be able to find something to replace it.

FAST FITNESS WORKOUTS

If you are new to regular exercise or haven't been active for some time then firstly congratulations on making a positive step to getting back into shape! Exercise is a great way to improve not just your body but also your mind.

Not only can regular physical activity help prevent illness it can also bring clarity and focus to your everyday life. It can help you lose weight, get trim and keep you feeling better. There are many benefits to reap from regular exercise.

Before starting on our Fast Fitness interval training workouts it is important to evaluate your basic level of fitness. If you have any major health concerns such as those listed below we recommend first seeking a health professionals advice.

- Heart disease
- Asthma or lung disease
- Type 1 or type 2 diabetes
- Kidney disease
- Arthritis

- Pain or discomfort in your chest
- Back pain
- Dizziness or lightheadedness
- Shortness of breath
- Ankle swelling

- Rapid heartbeat
- Smoker
- Overweight
- High blood pressure
- High Cholesterol

High Intensity Interval Training (HiiT), is a new kind of training program which concentrates on you giving your maximum effort through fast, intense bursts of exercise, followed by short recovery periods. It is quick and convenient and does not require equipment so you can do it anywhere, anytime.

These predominantly cardio exercises are designed to get your heart rate up, which in turn burns more fat in less time by increasing the body's need for oxygen during the effort. This creates an oxygen shortage, causing your body to ask for more oxygen during recovery. Often referred to as Excess Post-Exercise Oxygen Consumption (EPOC) this is the reason why concentrated exercise helps burn more fat and calories than traditional aerobic/cardio workouts.

Put simply regular high intensity workouts will help you increase your metabolism, reduce body fat and build lean muscle. In order to do this effectively our workouts should be combined with a healthy nutritional lifestyle, which is why the calorie counted slow cooker recipes in this book are the perfect partner. Physical and indeed everyday activities require energy to perform so we recommend a balanced diet of carbohydrates, protein and fat. Using a fitness tracker such as MyFitnessPal will help you achieve your daily nutritional needs.

Prior to performing any physical activity make sure you warm up first with some gentle stretching and exercises such as jogging on the spot and jumping jacks (see workouts from page 73). We have compiled 4 HiiT workouts to perform each week. To begin with ease yourself into these exercises especially if it has been some time since you have engaged in any cardio based training. As you progress and feel more comfortable with the routines you can increase intensity.

You should aim to do all 4 workouts within a 7 day period with rest days inbetween. Rest days are important as they give your body time to recover and repair - don't be tempted to skip them. Each workout lasts for approximately 15 minutes and a simple explanation with diagrams of how to correctly perform each exercise is provided. Over time, conditioning routines will help to make you lean in conjunction with a healthy balanced diet. They take work, time and dedication so be sure to stick at them and increase the intensity as the weeks go by.

As you progress you can, if you wish, start to introduce some basic weights (such as light dumbbells) into some of the exercises such as squats, lunges and standing mountain climbers. Taking just 15 mins out of your day to keep fit will set you on a lifelong path to a healthier, leaner and happier you.

WORKOUT TIPS

- Warm up and cool down before and after each workout
- Have a bottle of water to drink from between sets
- Remember to breathe through each exercise
- Keep your core tight & give maximum effort
- Focus on maintaining correct posture & form for each exercise

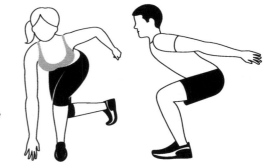

ABOUT 🍎 CookNation

CookNation is the leading publisher of innovative and practical recipe books for the modern, health conscious cook. CookNation titles bring together delicious, easy and practical recipes with their unique approach - easy and delicious, no-nonsense recipes - making cooking for diets and healthy eating fast, simple and fun.

With a range of #1 best-selling titles - from the innovative 'Skinny' calorie-counted series, to the 5:2 Diet Recipes collection - CookNation recipe books prove that 'Diet' can still mean 'Delicious'!

THE *Skinny*
SLOW COOKER
FAST FITNESS

RECIPE & WORKOUT BOOK

SOUPS UNDER 250 CALORIES

BEEF & NEW POTATO SOUP

220
calories per
serving

Ingredients

- 250g/9oz lean rump steak, finely sliced
- 1 leek, chopped
- 1 onion, chopped
- 2 garlic cloves, crushed
- 2 celery sticks, chopped
- 2 carrots, sliced lengthways
- 100g/4oz baby sweetcorn cobs, sliced lengthways
- 200g/7oz baby new potatoes, halved
- 1ltml/4 cups beef stock/broth
- Salt & pepper to taste
- Low cal cooking oil spray

Method

1 Preheat the slow cooker while you prepare the ingredients.

2 Gently sauté the leeks, onion, garlic & celery in a little low cal oil for a few minutes until they soften. Add all the ingredients to the slow cooker. Combine well, cover and leave to cook on high for 1½-2 hours or until the potatoes and steak are tender and cooked through. Check the seasoning and serve.

CHEFS NOTE

Any type of halved small or baby potatoes will work well for this recipe, but you could just use chunks of regular potatoes too.

PEA & HAM SOUP

245
calories per serving

Ingredients

- 1 onion, chopped
- 2 garlic cloves, crushed
- 150g/5oz pre soaked yellow split peas
- 2 carrots, chopped
- 2 tsp dried mixed herbs
- 125g/4oz smoked ham or gammon, chopped
- 1lt/4 cups chicken stock/broth
- Salt & pepper to taste
- Low cal cooking oil spray

Method

1 Preheat the slow cooker while you prepare the ingredients.

2 Gently sauté the onion & garlic in a little low cal oil for a few minutes until the onions soften. Add all the ingredients to the slow cooker. Combine well, cover and leave to cook on high for 1½-2 hours or until everything is tender. Remove 2 ladles of soup and use a blender to blend this to a smooth consistency. Return the blended portion of the soup to the rest of the soup. Combine well, season and serve.

CHEFS NOTE

Lean ham stripped from a smoked ham hock is ideal for this recipe, but you can use whatever you have to hand.

BEEF & VEGETABLE BROTH

Ingredients

- 1 leek, chopped
- 1 onion, chopped
- 2 garlic cloves, crushed
- 2 carrots, chopped
- 50g/2oz pre soaked pearl barley

- 2 celery sticks, chopped
- 225g/8oz lean rump steak, finely sliced
- 1ltml/4 cups beef stock/broth
- Salt & pepper to taste
- Low cal cooking oil spray

Method

1 Preheat the slow cooker while you prepare the ingredients.

2 Gently sauté the leeks, onion & garlic in a little low cal oil for a few minutes until they soften. Add all the ingredients to the slow cooker. Combine well, cover and leave to cook on high for 1½-2 hours or until the vegetables are tender and the steak is cooked through. Check the seasoning and serve.

CHEFS NOTE

Any cut of beef steak will work fine for this recipe provided it's sliced thinly enough.

CLASSIC CHICKEN SOUP

200 calories per serving

Ingredients

- 2 onions, chopped
- 2 carrots, finely chopped
- 2 sticks celery, finely chopped
- 2 garlic cloves, crushed
- 1lt/4 cups chicken stock/broth
- 350g/12oz cooked chicken breast, shredded
- Salt & pepper to taste
- Low cal cooking oil spray

Method

1 Preheat the slow cooker while you prepare the ingredients.

2 Gently sauté the onions, carrots, celery & garlic in a little low cal oil for a few minutes until the onions soften. Add all the ingredients to the slow cooker. Combine well, cover and leave to cook on high for 1-1½ hours or until the vegetables are tender. Remove 2 ladles of soup and use a blender to blend this to a smooth consistency. Return the blended portion to the rest of the soup. Stir well, season and serve.

CHEFS NOTE
Chicken soup is traditionally made with left over shredded chicken. This version uses the leanest cut of the bird - breast meat. Other cuts will have a higher fat content.

CHICKEN & MIXED BEAN SOUP

240 calories per serving

Ingredients

- 1 onion, chopped
- 2 garlic cloves, crushed
- 2 celery stalks, chopped
- 200g/7oz skinless chicken breast, chopped
- 1 red chilli, deseeded and chopped
- 1 carrot, chopped

- 200g/7oz tinned chopped tomatoes
- 400g/14oz tinned mixed beans, drained
- 1lt/4 cups chicken stock/broth
- 1 tbsp tomato puree/paste
- 1 tsp dried basil or oregano
- Salt & pepper to taste
- Low cal cooking oil spray

Method

1 Preheat the slow cooker while you prepare the ingredients.

2 Gently sauté the onion, garlic & celery in a little low cal oil for a few minutes until the onions soften. Add all the ingredients to the slow cooker. Combine well, cover and leave to cook on high for 1½-2 hours or until the chicken is cooked through. Season and serve.

CHEFS NOTE
This is a chunky soup which is should be left unblended. You could add a freshly chopped basil garnish if you like.

CHICKEN & FRESH ASPARAGUS SOUP

190 calories per serving

Ingredients

- 1 onion, chopped
- 2 garlic cloves, crushed
- 350g/12oz skinless chicken breast, finely sliced
- 50g/2oz fine rice noodles
- 120ml/½ cup dry white wine
- 1lt/4 cups chicken stock/broth
- 200g/7oz fresh asparagus tips, roughly chopped
- 1 small bunch spring onions/scallions, finely sliced lengthways
- Salt & pepper to taste
- Low cal cooking oil spray

Method

1 Preheat the slow cooker while you prepare the ingredients.

2 Gently sauté the onion & garlic in a little low cal oil for a few minutes until the onions soften. Add all the ingredients to the slow cooker, except the asparagus & spring onions. Combine well, cover and leave to cook on high for 1½ hours. Add the asparagus and cook for a further 10-20 minutes or until the chicken is cooked through and the asparagus is tender but not overcooked. Sprinkle with sliced spring onions, season and serve.

CHEFS NOTE
Adding the asparagus towards the end of the cooking time should ensure it still has a little crunch. Feel free to add at the beginning if you prefer it super-tender.

CHICKPEA & TOMATO SOUP

230 calories per serving

Ingredients

- 2 leeks, chopped
- 2 garlic cloves, crushed
- 125g/4oz courgettes/zucchini sliced
- 400g/14oz tinned chickpeas, drained
- 400g/14oz tinned chopped tomatoes
- 2 tbsp tomato puree/paste
- 500ml/2 cups vegetable stock/broth
- 125g/4oz tenderstem broccoli, roughly chopped
- Salt & pepper to taste
- Low cal cooking oil spray

Method

1 Preheat the slow cooker while you prepare the ingredients.

2 Gently sauté the leeks & garlic in a little low cal oil for a few minutes until the leeks soften. Add all the ingredients to the slow cooker. Combine well, cover and leave to cook on high for 1-1½ hours or until the vegetables are cooked through. Check the seasoning and serve.

CHEFS NOTE

Also known as garbanzo beans, chickpeas are a good source of protein.

BEETROOT SOUP

160 calories per serving

Ingredients

- 1 onion, chopped
- 1 tsp cumin seeds
- 150g/5oz potatoes, chopped
- 400g/14oz beetroot, cubed
- 750ml/3 cups vegetable stock/broth

- 1 tsp dried basil or oregano
- 1 tsp lemon juice
- 4 tbsp fat free Greek yoghurt
- Salt & pepper to taste
- Low cal cooking oil spray

Method

1 Preheat the slow cooker while you prepare the ingredients.

2 Gently sauté the onion & cumin seeds in a little low cal oil for a few minutes until the onions soften. Add all the ingredients to the slow cooker, except the Greek yoghurt. Combine well, cover and leave to cook on high for 1-1½ hours or until the vegetables are cooked through. Blend to a smooth consistency. Check the seasoning and serve with a dollop of yoghurt in the middle of each bowl.

CHEFS NOTE

This soup has a fantastic vibrant colour, which is contrasted by a generous dollop of white yoghurt.

SPANISH FISH SOUP

190 calories per serving

Ingredients

- 1 onion, chopped
- 2 garlic cloves, crushed
- 2 celery stalks, chopped
- 500g/1lb 2oz skinless boneless firm fish fillets/cubed
- 400g/14oz tinned chopped tomatoes
- 500ml/2 cups chicken or fish stock/broth
- 1 tsp each dried mixed herbs & paprika
- 2 tbsp tomato puree/paste
- Salt & pepper to taste
- Low cal cooking oil spray

Method

1 Preheat the slow cooker while you prepare the ingredients.

2 Gently sauté the onion, garlic & celery in a little low cal oil for a few minutes until the onions soften. Add all the ingredients to the slow cooker. Combine well, cover and leave to cook on high for 1-1½ hours or until the fish is cooked through. Season and serve.

CHEFS NOTE

If you don't have paprika you could add a little chilli instead.

THAI CRAB SOUP

210 calories per serving

Ingredients

- 400g/14oz tinned crab meat, drained
- 2 tbsp Thai red curry paste
- 750ml/3 cups chicken or fish stock/broth
- 250ml/1 cup low fat coconut milk
- Small bunch spring onions/scallions, chopped
- Salt & pepper to taste
- Low cal cooking oil spray

Method

1 Preheat the slow cooker while you prepare the ingredients.

2 Add all the ingredients to the slow cooker. Combine well, cover and leave to cook on high for 45mins-1 hour or until the soup is piping hot. Season and serve.

CHEFS NOTE

You could use fresh crab meat and/or prawns in this soup along with freshly chopped coriander/cilantro if you have it.

CREAMY CRAB & RICE SOUP

220
calories per serving

Ingredients

- 400g/14oz tinned crab meat, drained
- 100g/3½oz long grain rice
- 500ml/2 cups chicken or fish stock/broth
- 500ml/2 cups semi skimmed/half fat milk
- 1 tsp anchovy paste or 2 tsp Worcestershire sauce
- Salt & pepper to taste
- Low cal cooking oil spray

Method

1 Preheat the slow cooker while you prepare the ingredients.

2 Add all the ingredients to the slow cooker. Combine well, cover and leave to cook on high for 1-1½ hours or until the rice is tender. Blend to a smooth consistency, season and serve.

CHEFS NOTE
Use anchovy paste if you can as this will give a tasty additional depth to the soup.

THE *Skinny*
SLOW COOKER
FAST FITNESS

RECIPE & WORKOUT BOOK

MEALS UNDER 300 CALORIES

CORIANDER & SWEET POTATO CURRY

160 calories per serving

Ingredients

- 500g/1lb 2oz sweet potatoes, cubed
- 2 onions, finely chopped
- ½ tsp each turmeric, mild chilli powder, cumin, coriander/cilantro, paprika & salt
- 1 red chilli, finely chopped
- 2 carrots, sliced into batons
- 120ml/½ cup vegetable stock/broth
- 120ml/½ cup low fat coconut milk
- 2 tbsp freshly chopped coriander/cilantro
- Lime wedges to serve
- Salt & pepper to taste
- Low cal cooking oil spray

Method

1 Place all the ingredients in the slow cooker, except the coconut milk, chopped coriander & lime wedges. Combine well, cover and leave to cook on high for 3-5 hours or until the vegetables are tender and cooked through.

2 Add the coconut milk to the slow cooker. Gently stir through, sprinkle with chopped coriander and serve with the lime wedges.

CHEFS NOTE
Sweet potatoes are a fantastic versatile vegetable, which form the base of many Caribbean curries.

ALOO GOBI

Ingredients

- 1 large cauliflower head, split into florets
- ½ green cabbage, shredded
- 200g/7oz potatoes, cubed
- 400g/14oz tinned chopped tomatoes
- 2 garlic cloves, crushed
- 1 onion, chopped
- 1 tsp turmeric
- 2 tbsp tomato puree/paste

- ½ sp each cayenne pepper, cumin, coriander/cilantro, paprika, garam masala, salt & brown sugar
- 60ml/¼ cup vegetable stock/broth
- 2 tbsp chopped coriander/cilantro
- Salt & pepper to taste
- Low cal cooking oil spray

Method

1 Place all the ingredients in the slow cooker, except the chopped coriander. Combine well, cover and leave to cook on high for 3-5 hours or until the vegetables are tender and cooked through.

2 Sprinkle with chopped coriander and serve.

CHEFS NOTE
Spinach and broccoli make good additions to this dish too.

GINGER & FRESH TOMATO PRAWNS

160 calories per serving

Ingredients

- 500g/1lb 2oz raw, shelled king prawns
- 2 tsp freshly grated ginger
- ½ tsp each turmeric, cumin, coriander/cilantro, paprika, salt & brown sugar
- 1 red chilli, thinly sliced
- 2 garlic cloves, crushed

- 200g/7oz vine ripened tomatoes, roughly chopped
- 1 onion, sliced
- 2 tbsp tomato puree/paste
- Salt & pepper to taste
- Low cal cooking oil spray

Method

1 Mix the prawns, fresh ginger and turmeric together until the prawns are well covered.

2 Place all the ingredients in the slow cooker. Combine well, cover and leave to cook on high for 1-3 hours or until the prawns are cooked through.

CHEFS NOTE
If you don't have fresh ginger use a tsp ground ginger instead. You may choose to serve with a side dish depending on your diet.

PRAWN & SPICED FRESH PEAS

230 calories per serving

Ingredients

- 500g/1lb 2oz raw king prawns
- 200g/7oz fresh peas
- 200g/7oz vine ripened tomatoes, roughly chopped
- 2 garlic cloves, crushed
- 1 onion, chopped
- 120ml/½ cup tomato passata/sieved tomatoes

- ½ tsp each turmeric, cayenne pepper, cumin, coriander/cilantro, paprika, salt & brown sugar
- 2 tbsp tomato puree/paste
- 120ml/½ cup low fat coconut milk
- Salt & pepper to taste
- Low cal cooking oil spray

Method

1 Place all the ingredients in the slow cooker, except the coconut milk. Combine well, cover and leave to cook on high for 3-5 hours or until the prawns are cooked through.

2 Add the coconut milk to the slow cooker. Gently stir through and serve.

CHEFS NOTE
You could hold off adding the fresh peas until 30 mins before the end of cooking if you want them to have a little crunch.

COCONUT MILK MANGO CHICKEN

290 calories per serving

Ingredients

- 500g/1lb 2oz skinless chicken breast meat, cubed
- 2 onions, sliced
- 2 garlic cloves, crushed
- ½ tsp each turmeric, ground cumin & coriander/cilantro
- 2 tsp medium curry powder
- 2 tbsp tomato puree/paste
- 120ml/½ cup chicken stock/broth
- 120ml/½ cup low fat coconut milk
- 2 un-ripened mangos, peeled & de-stoned
- Salt & pepper to taste
- Low cal cooking oil spray

Method

1 Season the chicken and place in the slow cooker along with all the other ingredients except the coconut milk. Combine well, cover and leave to cook on high for 3-5 hours or until the chicken and mangoes are tender and cooked through.

2 Add the coconut milk to the slow cooker. Gently stir through and serve.

CHEFS NOTE
Ripe mangos are fine to use in this dish. Add them an hour before the end of cooking time so that they don't lose their form.

TAMARIND CHICKEN

260 calories per serving

Ingredients

- 500g/1lb 2oz skinless chicken breast meat, cubed
- 2 onions, sliced
- 2 garlic cloves, crushed
- ½ tsp each turmeric, ground cumin & coriander/cilantro
- 2 tsp medium curry powder
- 3 lemongrass stalks, finely chopped
- 2 tsp tamarind paste
- Juice & zest of 1 lime
- 3 curry leaves
- 200g/7oz spinach
- 2 tbsp tomato puree/paste
- 120ml/½ cup vegetable stock/broth
- 120ml/½ cup low fat coconut milk
- Salt & pepper to taste
- Low cal cooking oil spray

Method

1 Season the chicken and place in the slow cooker along with all the other ingredients except the coconut milk. Combine well, cover and leave to cook on high for 3-5 hours or until the chicken is tender and cooked through.

2 Add the coconut milk to the slow cooker. Gently stir through and serve.

CHEFS NOTE
Additional lime wedges make a nice garnish for this dish.

ALMOND CHICKEN

270 calories per serving

Ingredients

- 500g/1lb 2oz skinless chicken breast meat, cubed
- 2 onions, finely chopped
- 2 garlic cloves, crushed
- 1 tsp turmeric
- 1 tbsp ground almonds
- 1 tbsp tomato puree/paste

- ½ tsp each ground coriander/cilantro, cumin, paprika, mild chilli powder, ground ginger & salt
- 180ml/¾ cup chicken stock/broth
- 120ml/½ cup fat free Greek yoghurt
- Salt & pepper to taste
- Low cal cooking oil spray

Method

1 Season the chicken and quickly brown for a couple of minutes in a frying pan with a little low cal oil.

2 Remove from the heat and place in the slow cooker along with all the other ingredients except the Greek yoghurt. Combine well, cover and leave to cook on high for 3-5 hours or until the chicken is tender and cooked through.

3 Add the yoghurt to the slow cooker. Gently stir through and serve.

CHEFS NOTE
The almonds give this Korma style dish a lovely nutty taste.

FIERY CHICKEN CURRY

280 calories per serving

Ingredients

- 500g/1lb 2oz skinless chicken breast meat, cubed
- 2 tbsp tomato puree/paste
- 2 onions, finely chopped
- 2 garlic cloves, crushed
- 200g/7oz potatoes, diced
- 120ml/½ cup chicken stock/broth
- 250ml/1 cup tomato passata/sieved tomatoes
- ½ tsp each ground ginger, coriander/cilantro, turmeric, salt & cumin
- 2 tsp hot chilli powder & brown sugar
- Salt & pepper to taste
- Low cal cooking oil spray

Method

1 Season the chicken and place in the slow cooker along with all the other ingredients.

2 Combine well, cover and leave to cook on low for 6-7 hours or until the chicken is tender and cooked through.

CHEFS NOTE
You could also use cayenne pepper rather than hot chilli powder for this recipe.

THAI BASIL PORK

280 calories per serving

Ingredients

- 500g/1lb 2oz pork tenderloin, cubed
- 2 onions, finely chopped
- 2 tbsp Thai red curry paste
- 2 tsp tamarind paste
- ½ tsp ground coriander/cilantro
- 1 red pepper, sliced
- 2 carrots, sliced into batons
- 1 lemongrass stalk, finely chopped
- 3 tbsp freshly chopped basil
- 500ml/2 cups chicken stock/broth
- Salt & pepper to taste
- Low cal cooking oil spray

Method

1 Season the pork and quickly brown for a couple of minutes in a frying pan with a little low cal oil.

2 Remove from the heat and place in the slow cooker along with all the other ingredients. Combine well, cover and leave to cook on low for 5-7 hours or until the pork is tender and cooked through.

CHEFS NOTE
Lean pork is a great source of protein, is low in fat and contains important B nutrients - thiamine and niacin - which help protect against heart attacks and strokes.

FISH STEW

245 calories per serving

Ingredients

- 450g/1lb white fish fillets, cubed
- 1 leek, chopped
- 4 garlic cloves, crushed
- 1 400g/14oz tin chopped tomatoes
- 100g/3 ½oz frozen peas
- 2 stalk celery, chopped
- 1 onion chopped
- ½ tsp fennel seeds
- 1 tbsp dried basil
- 1lt/4 cups fish stock/broth
- 250g/9oz raw prawns
- Salt & Pepper to taste

Method

1 Mix together all the ingredients, except the fish, peas and prawns in the slow cooker. Season, cover and leave to cook on low for 4-5 hours or high for 2-3 hours.

2 Meanwhile season the fish and prawns. 45 mins before the end of cooking add the fish, prawns and peas. Continue to cook until the seafood is cooked right through and the peas are tender.

3 Serve with noodles as a soup stew.

CHEFS NOTE

Feel free to use any type of meaty white fish you like and, if you feel adventurous, you could add some squid, octopus or clams to the stew.

CORIANDER & GARLIC PRAWNS

269 calories per serving

Ingredients

- 500g/1lb2oz raw king prawns
- 200g/7oz frozen peas
- 1 tsp sunflower oil
- 2 onions, sliced
- 200g/8oz cherry tomatoes, halved
- 1 tsp ground ginger
- 4 garlic cloves, crushed
- 3 tbsp curry paste
- 2 tbsp fresh chopped coriander/cilantro
- 250ml/1 cup passata/sieved tomatoes
- Salt & pepper to taste

Method

1 Add all the ingredients to the slow cooker, cover and leave to cook on low for 1-2 hours or until the prawns are cooked through and the peas are tender.

2 Sprinkle with chopped coriander and serve with rice.

CHEFS NOTE
This is a really simple 'cheat' curry using curry paste. If you want a slightly different taste you could use less passatta and add a little coconut milk to the recipe after cooking.

TUNA & NOODLE CATTIA

250
calories per
serving

Ingredients

- 350g/12oz fresh egg noodles
- 1 onion, chopped
- 1 400/14oz tin fat free condensed mushroom soup
- 100g/3 ½oz frozen peas
- 2 200g/7oz tins tuna steaks or flakes in water
- 1 tsp garlic powder
- Salt & pepper to taste
- Pinch of crushed chilli flakes

Method

1 Quickly cook the pasta or noodles in salted boiling water. Save 3 tbsp of the drained water and then combine it along with all the other ingredients in the slow cooker. Cover and leave to cook on low for 1½ hours.

2 This is lovely served with a sliced red onion & tomato salad with a little Parmesan.

CHEFS NOTE

An absolute classic American slow cooker recipe, Tuna & Noodle casserole is always a winner. It's also a favourite for for a post workout meal.

SWEET & CITRUS SALMON

270 calories per serving

Ingredients

- 500g/1lb 2oz thick boneless salmon fillets
- 1 onion, chopped
- 1 tbsp light soy sauce
- Juice of 2 fresh limes or 3 tbsp lime juice
- 2 garlic cloves, crushed
- 1 tsp sugar dissolved into 3 tbsp warm water and brushed onto the fillets
- Low cal cooking spray
- Salt & pepper to taste

Method

1 Chop the onion and sauté for a couple of minutes with the garlic in a little low cal oil. Remove from the pan and carefully combine all the ingredients in the slow cooker.

2 Cook on low for 1½ hours with the lid tightly on.

3 Check your fish is properly cooked by flaking it a little with a fork and serve with salad potatoes and carrots. Alternatively use in a lovely warm salad served with a little crusty bread.

CHEFS NOTE

Salmon can be relatively expensive so you can substitute for Tilapia, Basa or talk to your fishmonger for recommendations.

GREEN THAI FISH CURRY

215 calories per serving

Ingredients

- 500g/1lb 2oz meaty white fish fillets (go for whatever is on sale) haddock, cod, pollock, cobbler
- 3 onions, chopped
- 1 tsp fresh ginger or ½ tsp ground ginger
- 3 cloves garlic crushed
- 1 whole red chilli, chopped
- 50g/2oz watercress
- 2 tbsp Thai green curry paste
- 500ml/2 cups low fat coconut milk
- Low cal cooking spray
- Salt & pepper to taste

Method

1 Sauté the onions & green beans with the ginger and garlic over a low heat in a little low cal spray.

2 Season the fish fillets with salt and pepper and carefully combine all the ingredients (except the watercress) in the slow cooker.

3 Cook on low for 1½ hours with the lid tightly shut. This timing should mean your fish is not overcooked and the green beans have some bite to them.

4 Check the fish is properly cooked through by flaking it a little with a fork and gently add the watercress salad to the mix before serving. Serve with noodles or rice.

CHEFS NOTE
Compared to meat, fish cooks more quickly in the slow cooker and as such fish recipes can be really handy if you haven't got too much cooking time. This recipe is a fantastic and easy Thai curry that is simple to prep and doesn't take long at all in the slow cooker.

SWEET & SOUR PINEAPPLE PORK

238 calories per serving

Ingredients

- 900g/2lb lean cubed pork
- 1 tbsp plain/all purpose flour
- 1 400g/14oz tin pineapple chunks (reserve the juice)
- 1 onion, chopped
- 1 green (bell) pepper, chopped
- 2 carrots, cut into batons

- 1 tbsp brown sugar
- ½ tsp salt
- 2 tbsp lime juice
- 1 tbsp light soy sauce
- 120ml/ ½ cup boiling water
- Low cal cooking spray

Method

1 Brown the pork in a frying pan with a little low cal spray. Remove the pork and dust with the flour.

2 Put all the other ingredients except the pineapple chunks into the slow cooker (include the pineapple juice).

3 Combine everything and leave to cook on low for 4-5 hours with the lid tightly closed. Check the pork is tender and then add the pineapple chunks. Leave for a further 30 min and serve with boiled rice.

CHEFS NOTE

Sweet and Sour is one of the most loved Chinese meals in the world. This is not supposed to be an authentic copy, just take it as a super simple replica which should satisfy your eastern cravings!

BUDAPEST'S BEST BEEF GOULASH

228 calories per serving

Ingredients

- 900g/2lb lean stewing beef cut into chunks (trim off any fat)
- 1 red (bell) pepper, sliced
- 3 cloves garlic, crushed
- 250ml/1 cup beef stock/broth or boiling water
- 220ml/ 1 cup red wine (if you have some)

- 1 400g/14oz tin chopped tomatoes
- 1 tbsp tomato puree/paste
- 1 tsp paprika
- 1 ½ tbsp plain/all purpose flour
- 1 onion, chopped
- Low cal cooking spray
- Salt & pepper to taste

Method

1 Season the beef and quickly brown in a smoking hot pan with a little low cal spray. Remove from pan and dust with the flour (the easiest way is to put the beef and flour into a plastic bag and give it a good shake).

2 Add all the ingredients to the slow cooker and combine well. Leave to cook on low with the lid tightly shut for 5-6 hours or until the beef is tender and cooked through. If you want to thicken up a little, leave to cook for a further 45 mins with the lid off.

3 Lovely with a salad & some crusty bread or serve with sour cream and tagliatelle pasta.

CHEFS NOTE
Goulash is a European dish which suits the slow cooker beautifully. After hours of gentle cooking, this 'tougher' meat becomes a tender cut that just melts in the mouth.

SWEET ASIAN CHICKEN

256 calories per serving

Ingredients

- 500g/1lb 2oz skinless chicken breasts
- 2 garlic cloves, crushed
- 1 onion, chopped
- 60ml/¼ cup runny honey
- 2 tbsp tomato puree/paste
- 4 tbsp light soy sauce
- 2 carrots cut into batons
- Pinch crushed chilli
- 250ml/1 cup fresh orange juice
- 1 tsp sunflower oil
- 1 tsp cornstarch dissolved in a little water to form a thick paste

Method

1 Combine all the ingredients in a bowl and add to the slow cooker. Cook on low for 5-6 hours or on high for 3-4 hours with the lid tightly shut or until the chicken is cooked through and tender. Add a little water during cooking if needed.

2 Serve with fine egg noodles or rice. If you want to add a little extra touch add a garnish of spring onions & sesame seeds.

CHEFS NOTE

The honey, soy and orange juice in this dish make it a hit with the kids and adds a little eastern flavor to excite evening meal times.

ZINGY LIME CHICKEN

200 calories per serving

Ingredients

- 500g/1lb 2oz skinless chicken breasts
- Juice 2 limes or 3 ½ tablespoons bottled lime juice
- Bunch fresh coriander/cilantro chopped and some to garnish
- 1 sliced green chilli, sliced (or a pinch of dried chilli flakes)
- 16oz/450g salsa (jar)

Or make your own salsa:
- Combine 1 chopped onion, 1 clove crushed garlic, 1 chopped green chilli to 2 x tins 400g/14oz chopped tomatoes + sea salt to taste
- 4 tsp your favourite packet taco seasoning

Method

1 Put everything together in the slow cooker making sure the chicken is covered with the rest of the ingredients. With the lid tightly shut leave to cook for 4-5 hours on high or 6-8 hours on the low setting.

2 Ensure the chicken is cooked through and tender then shred it a little with 2 forks and serve with a fresh green salad/rice or quesadillas (flour tortilla).

CHEFS NOTE

Packed with protein, skinless chicken breast is a fantastic low fat meat to use in the slow cooker. The citrus lightness of this recipe is perfect for summer months as well as a welcome taste bud infusion during the cold seasons.

LOVELY LEMONY GARLICKY CHICKEN

208 calories per serving

Ingredients

- 500g/1lb 2oz skinless chicken breasts
- 3 garlic cloves, crushed
- 3 tbsp lemon juice
- 1 onion, chopped
- 1 tsp runny honey

- 1 tsp cornstarch dissolved in a little warm water to make a paste
- 500ml/2 cups chicken stock/broth
- Salt & pepper to taste
- Bunch fresh basil

Method

1 Combine all the ingredients in the slow cooker and leave to cook on low for 5-6 hours or on high 3-4 hours with the lid tightly shut.

2 Ensure the chicken is cooked through and tender, and serve with steamed vegetables and rice.

CHEFS NOTE

This is a really simple protein-packed dish that really benefits from using fresh basil.

THE *Skinny*
SLOW COOKER
FAST FITNESS

RECIPE & WORKOUT BOOK

MEALS UNDER 400 CALORIES

SMOKY PINTO BEANS & FRESH SPRING ONIONS

310 calories per serving

Ingredients

- 1 large bunch spring onions
- 3 tbsp freshly chopped flat leaf parsley
- 1kg/2¼lb tinned pinto beans, drained & rinsed
- 1 tbsp tomato puree/paste
- 2 tsp brown sugar

- 200g/7oz shop bought roasted peppers, roughly chopped
- 120ml/½ cup vegetable stock/broth
- 1 tbsp smoked paprika
- 1 garlic clove, crushed
- Salt & pepper to taste

Method

1 Slice the spring onions diagonally, mix with the chopped parsley and put to one side.

2 Add the drained pinto beans, puree, sugar, peppers, stock, paprika & garlic to the slow cooker. Cover and leave to cook on high for 2-4 hours or until the stock has reduced and the smoky beans are tender.

3 Remove from the slow cooker and divide into bowls. Check the seasoning, sprinkle with the fresh parsley & spring onion mix and serve.

CHEFS NOTE
Pinto beans are a staple of Mexican cooking. Garnishing with fresh spring onions gives this dish a light crunchy bite.

SWEET & SPICY CHICKEN WINGS

350
calories per serving

Ingredients

- 15 skinless, chicken wings
- 2 tbsp runny honey
- 1 tsp English mustard
- 3 garlic cloves, crushed
- 3 tbsp Worcestershire sauce

- A large bunch spring onions/scallions, finely chopped
- Low cal cooking oil spray
- Salt & pepper to taste

Method

1 First pierce the wings with a fork or skewer. Mix together the honey, mustard, garlic & Worcestershire sauce and brush all over the wings.

2 Place in the slow cooker with a little low cal spray, cover and leave to cook on high for 2-3 hours or until the chicken is cooked through and piping hot.

3 Sprinkle with finely chopped spring onions and serve.

CHEFS NOTE
These wings are delicious served with homemade coleslaw, but be careful not to make it too calorific.

SPICED LAMB SKEWERS

320 calories per serving

Ingredients

- 500g/1lb 2oz lean lamb fillet
- ½ tsp each ground cumin, ginger & paprika
- 2 garlic cloves, crushed
- 12 cherry tomatoes
- 12 button mushrooms
- 2 tbsp freshly chopped coriander/cilantro
- 4 tbsp fat free Greek yoghurt
- 8 skewers
- Low cal cooking oil spray
- Salt & pepper to taste

Method

1 First brown the lamb in a frying pan on a high heat with a little low cal oil for a minute or two to seal the meat. Remove from the pan and place in a bowl with the whole tomatoes & mushrooms. Sprinkle the cumin, ginger, paprika & crushed garlic into the bowl and combine really well.

2 Season and pierce the lamb, tomatoes and mushrooms in turn onto the skewers. Spray with a little oil and place in the slow cooker. Cover and leave to cook on high for 2-4 hours or until the lamb is cooked to your liking.

3 Sprinkle with chopped coriander and serve with a dollop of Greek yoghurt for dipping.

CHEFS NOTE
Be sure not to overcook the lamb as you don't want it to be tough.

BBQ SHREDDED BEEF

375
calories per serving

Ingredients

- 2 tbsp brown sugar
- 2 tbsp tomato puree/paste
- 2 onions, sliced
- 2 tbsp Dijon mustard
- 2 tbsp Worcestershire sauce
- 2 tbsp white wine vinegar

- 1 tsp paprika
- 3 garlic cloves crushed
- 120ml/½ cup tomato passata/paste
- 600g/1lb 5oz lean beef stewing steak, cubed
- Salt & pepper to taste

Method

1 First place all the ingredients, except the stewing steak in a saucepan. Bring to the boil and reduce to a gentle simmer. Allow to cook for 8-10 minutes.

2 Place in a blender and blitz into a smooth BBQ sauce. Check the seasoning and place the beef and BBQ sauce in the slow cooker. Cover and leave to cook on low for 8-10 hours or until the beef is meltingly tender (add a little water during cooking if you think the dish needs it).

3 Remove from the slow cooker and use 2 forks to shred. Check the seasoning and serve.

CHEFS NOTE
This shredded BBQ beef is a perfect low maintenance addition to a family BBQ that you can prepare ahead of time.

PANCETTA RISOTTO

340 calories per serving

Ingredients

- 75g/3oz pancetta bacon, trimmed & diced
- 1 onion, sliced
- 1 garlic clove, crushed
- 300g/11oz Arborio risotto rice
- 1lt/4 cups chicken stock/broth
- 200g/7oz rocket
- Low cal cooking oil spray
- Salt & pepper to taste

Method

1 First sauté the pancetta, onion & garlic in a little low cal oil for a few minutes. Remove from the pan and chop as finely as possible. Return to the pan and add the rice. Stir around well to coat the rice in the residual oil.

2 Place the contents of the pan in the slow cooker along with the stock. Combine well, cover and leave to cook on low for approx 2 hours or until the stock has been absorbed.

3 Check the rice; if it is not tender add some more stock and leave to cook for a little longer. When the risotto is tender and the stock has been absorbed, season and serve with the rocket.

CHEFS NOTE
Chopping the sautéed pancetta and onions as small as possible means their lovely salty sweet flavour will permeate every mouthful of this lovely risotto.

LEAN MINI MEATBALLS & FRESH HERBS

375 calories per serving

Ingredients

- 200g/7oz lean turkey mince
- 1 garlic clove
- 2 tbsp fresh breadcrumbs
- 2 tbsp mixed fresh herbs (basil, parsley & rosemary is a good mix)
- 400g/14oz tinned chopped tomatoes
- 2 tbsp tomato puree/paste
- ½ tsp brown sugar
- 300g/11oz spaghetti
- Salt & pepper to taste

Method

1 Place the turkey mince, garlic, breadcrumbs & fresh herbs in a food processor. Pulse for a few seconds to combine and use your hands to form the meat mixture into tiny meatballs about 2/3cm in diameter.

2 Add meatballs, chopped tomatoes, puree and sugar to the slow cooker. Combine well, cover and leave to cook on low for 4-6 hours or until the meatballs are cooked through and the sauce is thickened.

3 Meanwhile cook the spaghetti in salted boiling water until tender. Drain the pasta and divide into bowls. Load the meatballs and sauce on top and serve.

CHEFS NOTE
To make fresh breadcrumbs just put a slice of bread in the food processor and whizz for a few seconds.

SUMMER SQUASH & CHILLI LINGUINE

310 calories per serving

Ingredients

- 1 butternut squash, peeled, deseeded & cubed
- 1 onion, sliced
- 1 red chilli, sliced
- 1 garlic clove, crushed
- 120ml/½ cup vegetable stock/broth
- 2 tbsp low fat crème fraiche
- 300g/11oz linguine pasta
- Low cal cooking oil spray
- Salt & pepper to taste

Method

1 Add the squash, onion, chilli, garlic & vegetable stock to the slow cooker. Combine well, cover and leave to cook on low for 3-4 hours or until the squash is tender.

2 Cook the linguine pasta in salted boiling water until tender. Take everything out of the slow cooker and place in a food processor. Add the crème fraiche and blitz until smooth. Toss with the drained linguine, season and serve.

CHEFS NOTE
Add a little more boiling water or stock if you feel the pasta sauce is a little thick when blending.

MOROCCAN LAMB & APRICOT CURRY

360 calories per serving

Ingredients

- 500g/1lb 2oz lean lamb fillet, cubed
- 2 onions, finely chopped
- 2 garlic cloves, crushed
- 400g/14oz fresh chopped tomatoes
- 100g/3½oz dried apricots, finely chopped
- 2 carrots, sliced into batons
- ½ tsp each ground ginger, turmeric, coriander/cilantro & paprika
- A pinch each of ground cinnamon, nutmeg & salt
- 120ml/½ cup vegetable stock/broth
- Salt & pepper to taste
- Low cal cooking oil spray

Method

1 Season the lamb and quickly brown for a couple of minutes in a frying pan with a little low cal oil.

2 Remove from the heat and place in the slow cooker along with all the other ingredients. Combine well, cover and leave to cook on low for 5-7 hours or until the lamb is tender and cooked through.

CHEFS NOTE
Make sure the lamb is trimmed of as much visible fat as possible.

KOREAN BEEF & POTATO CURRY

320 calories per serving

Ingredients

- 500g/1lb 2oz lean beef stewing steak
- 2 onions, sliced
- 2 garlic cloves, crushed
- 1 tsp turmeric
- ½ tsp each ground cumin, coriander/ cilantro, hot chilli powder & paprika
- A pinch of ground ginger, salt & garam masala

- 200g/7oz new potatoes, thickly sliced
- 200g/7oz spinach leaves
- 200g/7oz vine ripened tomatoes, roughly chopped
- 120ml/½ cup beef stock/broth
- 1 tbsp tomato puree/paste
- Salt & pepper to taste
- Low cal cooking oil spray

Method

1 Season the beef and quickly brown for a couple of minutes in a frying pan with a little low cal oil.

2 Remove from the heat and place in the slow cooker along with all the other ingredients. Combine well, cover and leave to cook on low for 6-8 hours or until the beef is tender and cooked through.

CHEFS NOTE
Tinned chopped tomatoes are also fine for this recipe if you don't have fresh tomatoes to hand.

CARIBBEAN BEEF CURRY

340 calories per serving

Ingredients

- 500g/1lb 2oz lean beef stewing steak, cubed
- 1 tbsp hot curry powder
- 1 red chilli, finely chopped
- 1 tbsp tomato puree/paste
- 400g/14oz tinned chopped tomatoes
- 2 onions, sliced
- 3 garlic cloves, crushed
- 1 tbsp dried thyme
- 150g/5oz sweet potato, diced
- 60ml/¼ cup beef stock/broth
- 1 tbsp coconut cream
- Salt & pepper to taste
- Low cal cooking oil spray

Method

1 Season the steak and quickly brown for a couple of minutes in a frying pan with a little low cal oil.

2 Remove from the heat and place in the slow cooker along with all the other ingredients except the coconut cream. Combine well, cover and leave to cook on low for 6-8 hours or until the beef is tender and cooked through.

3 Add the coconut cream to the slow cooker. Gently stir through and serve

CHEFS NOTE
This curry is also nice with a little mixed spice added to give a fragrant finish to the dish.

SAUSAGE & SPINACH WITH GNOCCHI

309 calories per serving

Ingredients

- 6 pork or beef sausages (skins removed)
- 250ml/1 cup tomato passata/sieved tomatoes
- 1 tsp dried rosemary
- 1 splash red wine vinegar

- ½ tsp salt
- 200g/7oz tinned chopped tomatoes
- 100g/3 ½ oz fresh spinach
- 1 bunch fresh spinach
- 1 lb 2 oz / 500 g packet gnocchi

Method

1 Brown the sausage meat in a frying pan and break up well. Add all the ingredients except the gnocchi and spinach to the slow cooker and combine. Close the lid tightly and leave to cook on high for 3-4 hours.

2 When the meat is well cooked stir in the fresh spinach & gnocchi and leave to cook for a further 10-20 mins or until the gnocchi is tender.

CHEFS NOTE

This lovely recipe uses sausage meat to create a thick, luxurious sauce which is just perfect with freshly cooked gnocchi. You can also add some crushed chilli if you want a bit of heat.

ALMONDS, BEEF & OLIVES

392 calories per serving

Ingredients

- 600g/1lb 5oz lean stewing steak/chuck steak, cubed
- 250ml/1 cup beef stock/broth
- 60ml/¼ cup red wine
- 1 tbsp plain/all purpose flour
- 1 tsp each smoked paprika, dried basil & rosemary
- 200g/7oz pitted olives
- 25g/1oz chopped almonds
- Salt & pepper to taste

Method

1 Season the beef and coat well in the plain flour. Add all the ingredients, except the olives, to the slow cooker and leave to cook on low for 4-6 hours or until the beef is tender.

2 Add a little more stock or wine during cooking if needed and adjust the seasoning. 20 minutes before the end of cooking add the olives, warm through and serve.

CHEFS NOTE
This dish is delicious served with creamed spinach and/or honeyed carrots. Feel free to use a different mix of dried herbs to suit your taste. You can also add a tablespoon of tomato puree during cooking to thicken if you prefer.

RAGU A LA BOLOGNESE

344 calories per serving

Ingredients

- 500g/1lb 2oz lean minced/ground beef
- 1 400g/14oz tin chopped tomatoes
- 250ml/1 cup passata/sieved tomatoes
- 1 tsp each dried oregano & thyme
- 1 stick celery, chopped
- 2 bay leaves
- 1 tbsp tomato puree/paste
- 3 garlic cloves, crushed
- 2 onions, chopped
- Salt and pepper to taste
- Low cal cooking spray

Method

1 Quickly brown the meat in a frying pan with a little low cal spray.

2 Combine all the ingredients in the slow cooker and close the lid tightly. Leave to cook on low for 5-6 hours or high 3-4 hours. Make sure the meat is cooked through and serve with rigatoni, penne or spaghetti.

CHEFS NOTE

Nothing is simpler or more satisfying than Spaghetti Bolognese. You can add mushrooms and peppers to the recipe if you like, plus a dash or two of Worcestershire sauce gives extra depth.

SLOW SCOTTISH STOVIES

333
calories per
serving

Ingredients

- 175g/6oz potatoes, diced
- 2 large onions, chopped
- 250ml/1 cup vegetable stock/broth
- 450g/1lb left over roast beef (or other cooked red meat)
- Salt & pepper to taste

Method

1 Combine all the ingredients together in the slow cooker and cook on low for 5-6 hours or on high 3-4 hours with the lid tightly shut. The liquid should all be gone by the end of the cooking time, if it hasn't, remove the lid and leave to cook for a little longer.

2 Stir through and serve in bowls with British brown sauce if you have some!

CHEFS NOTE

This is a great recipe to use up any cooked left-over red meat you might have. Traditionally it is served with plain Scottish oatcakes and it's super simple to make. Perfect for a carb rich post workout meal.

CHICKEN & ALMONDS

Ingredients

- 500g/1lb 2oz skinless chicken breasts, cut into chunks
- 1 tbsp ground almonds
- ½ tsp paprika
- 2 red (bell) peppers, sliced
- 1 onion, chopped
- 2 cloves garlic, crushed
- 1 tbsp white wine vinegar
- 2 tbsp chopped flat leaf parsley
- 1 400g/14oz chopped tomatoes
- 300g/11oz tinned haricot beans, drained
- ½ tsp dried chilli flakes
- 100g/3½oz frozen peas
- Low cal cooking spray
- Salt & pepper to taste

Method

1 Brown the chicken pieces in a little low cal spray. Add all the ingredients, except the parsley, into the slow cooker.

2 Season, cover and leave to cook on high for 3-4 hours or low for 5-6 hours.

3 Sprinkle with chopped parsley and serve with rice and/or crusty bread.

CHEFS NOTE
This Spanish inspired dish is great as a main meal but can also be served as a delicious ciabatta topping.

THE *Skinny*
SLOW COOKER
FAST FITNESS

RECIPE & WORKOUT BOOK

MEALS UNDER 500 CALORIES

BASIL 'PESTO' LINGUINI

450 calories per serving

Ingredients

- 1 handful pine nuts
- 2 garlic cloves
- 1 tbsp parmesan cheese
- 1 tsp rock salt
- 2 tbsp lemon juice
- 1 large bunch basil leaves

- 150g/5oz asparagus tips, roughly chopped
- 250g/9oz portabella mushrooms, sliced
- 60ml/ ¼ cup vegetable stock/broth
- 300g/11oz linguine
- 2 tbsp low fat crème fraiche
- Salt & pepper to taste

Method

1 Add the pine nuts, garlic cloves, parmesan cheese, salt & lemon juice to a food processor and pulse to a fine mixture. Place all the ingredients, except the linguine & crème fraiche in the slow cooker. Combine gently, cover and leave to cook on high for 1-2 hours or until the vegetables are tender.

2 Meanwhile cook the linguine in salted boiling water until tender. Toss the cooked vegetables and linguine together along with the crème fraiche. Season well and serve.

CHEFS NOTE

This is not a true pesto but it's a lighter olive oil-free alternative. Adjust the salt, lemon and garlic to your own taste.

CARAMELISED GINGER SWEET POTATOES

445 calories per serving

Ingredients

- 1kg/2¼lb sweet potatoes, cubed
- 1 tbsp olive oil
- 2 tbsp water
- 2 garlic cloves, crushed
- 1 onion, sliced
- 1 tbsp freshly grated ginger
- 1 tbsp brown sugar
- 1 tsp each paprika & all spice
- Salt & pepper to taste

Method

1 Place all the ingredients in the slow cooker,

2 Combine well, season, cover and leave to cook on high for 2-4 hours or until the potatoes are tender. Season and serve.

CHEFS NOTE
These sweet potatoes are delicious. Make sure they don't 'burn' by stirring and adding a little more water to the slow cooker during cooking if needed.

MEXICAN ONIONS & KIDNEY BEANS

420 calories per serving

Ingredients

- 3 large onions, sliced
- 3 garlic cloves, crushed
- 1 tbsp olive oil
- 1 tbsp paprika
- 1 tsp cumin
- 1 tbsp sweet chilli sauce
- 100g/7oz potatoes, chopped
- 400g/14oz tinned kidney beans, rinsed

- 200g/7oz mushrooms
- 3 tbsp tomato puree/paste
- 250ml/1 cup tomato passata/sieved tomatoes
- 4 tbsp fat free Greek yoghurt
- 2 tbsp freshly chopped coriander/cilantro
- Salt & pepper to taste

Method

1 Gently sauté the onions and garlic in the olive oil for a few minutes. Mix the paprika and cumin with a little warm water to make a paste and stir this through the onions. Continue to cook for a minute or two, add the sweet chilli sauce and combine well.

2 Place all the ingredients, except the yoghurt and chopped coriander, in the slow cooker. Stir, season, cover and leave to cook on high for 1-3 hours or until all the vegetables are tender. Serve in shallow bowls with a tbsp of yoghurt on the top of each bowl, sprinkled with fresh coriander.

CHEFS NOTE
Feel free to spice this dish up further with fresh chopped chillies or ground cayenne pepper.

HIGHLAND VENISON STEW

400 calories per serving

Ingredients

- 500g/1lb 2oz venison stewing steak, cubed
- 1 tbsp plain/all purpose flour
- ½ tsp ground all spice
- 2 carrots, chopped
- 1 garlic clove, crushed
- 1 onion, sliced

- 2 celery stalks, sliced
- 380ml/1½ cups chicken stock/broth
- 2 tbsp worcestershire sauce
- 300g/11oz tenderstem broccoli spears
- 300g/11oz new potatoes, sliced
- Low cal cooking oil spray
- Salt & pepper to taste

Method

1 Season the venison and brown in a hot frying pan with a little low cal oil for a few minutes. Remove from the pan and place in a small plastic bag with the flour and all spice. Shake well to cover each piece of venison in flour.

2 Place the floured meat in the slow cooker along with all the other ingredients. Cover and leave to cook on high for 4-6 hours or until the venison is tender and cooked through. Season and serve.

CHEFS NOTE

Venison is a tasty and lean game meat which is now readily available in most supermarkets.

BEST BEEF TACOS

420 calories per serving

Ingredients

- 500g/1lb 2oz lean minced/ground beef
- 1 garlic clove, crushed
- 2 onions, sliced
- 1 tsp each cumin, paprika & cayenne pepper
- ½ tsp ground ginger
- 1 red (bell) pepper, finely chopped
- 2 tbsp worcestershire sauce
- 2 tbsp tomato puree/paste
- 400g/14oz tinned chopped tomatoes
- 8 Old El Paso taco shells
- 4 tbsp fat free Greek yoghurt
- 2 romaine lettuces, shredded
- Salt & pepper to taste

Method

1 Place all the ingredients, except the taco shells, yoghurt & lettuce, in the slow cooker. Combine well, cover and leave to cook on high for 4-6 hours or until the mince is tender and cooked through.

2 Serve the mince in taco shells with yoghurt and shredded lettuce on the top.

CHEFS NOTE
Grated cheese is good on tacos too but it will increase the calorie count - so don't overdo it!

PAPRIKA PORK GOULASH

400 calories per serving

Ingredients

- 500g/1lb 2oz pork tenderloin, cubed
- 2 red (bell) peppers, sliced
- 1 onion, sliced
- 2 garlic cloves, crushed
- 2 tbsp paprika
- ½ tsp cayenne pepper
- ½ tsp each salt & brown sugar
- 250ml/1 cup tomato passata/sieved tomatoes
- 60ml/¼cup chicken stock/broth
- 200g/7oz long grain rice
- 2 tbsp fat free Greek yoghurt
- Low cal cooking oil spray
- Salt & pepper to taste

Method

1 Season the pork tenderloin.

2 Gently sauté the peppers, onions & garlic in a little low cal spray for a few minutes until softened. Add all the ingredients, except the rice and yoghurt, to the slow cooker. Cover and leave to cook on high for 4-6 hours or until the pork is cooked through. At the end of the cooking time stir the yoghurt through.

3 Meanwhile cook the rice in salted boiling water until tender. Drain and serve as a bed for the pork.

CHEFS NOTE
Paprika is a lovely gently 'warming' spice, whilst the cayenne pepper adds the 'kick'.

MELTING BEEF TOPSIDE & SPINACH

460 calories per serving

Ingredients

- 1kg/2¼lb piece lean beef topside
- 3 carrots, chopped
- 2 onions, chopped
- 2 parsnips, chopped
- 1 celery stalk, chopped
- 1 tbsp olive oil
- ½ tsp ground cinnamon
- 1 tsp each ground coriander/cilantro, thyme & salt
- 500ml/2 cups chicken stock/broth
- 400g/14oz spinach
- 1 large bunch freshly chopped flat leaf parsley
- Salt & pepper to taste

Method

1 Trim the beef of any visible fat and season well with salt & pepper.

2 Gently sauté the carrots, onions, parsnips and celery in the olive oil for a few minutes until softened. Add the coriander, thyme, salt & cinnamon and stir well. Put the sautéed vegetables, beef and stock into the slow cooker. Cover and leave to cook on low for 8-10 hours or until the beef is meltingly tender. Add the spinach to the slow cooker and cook for 10-20 minutes or until the spinach gently wilts.

3 Remove the beef from the slow cooker. Slice thinly and arrange on plates with the chopped vegetables and wilted spinach. Sprinkle with chopped parsley and serve.

CHEFS NOTE
If parsnips are out of season try substituting with sweet potato.

SPINACH & LAMB STEW

467 calories per serving

Ingredients

- 500g/1lb 2oz lean lamb cut into bite sized chunks (any lean cut will work)
- 2 cloves garlic, crushed
- Zest of 1 lemon
- 1 onion, chopped
- 2 400g/14oz tins chopped tomatoes
- 1 tbsp tomato puree/paste
- 1 400g/14oz tin chickpeas, drained
- 400g/14oz fresh spinach, chopped

Dried herb mix of the following:
- 1 tsp coriander/cilantro
- 1 tsp turmeric
- ½ tsp cumin
- ½ tsp black pepper
- ½ tsp oregano
- 2 tbsp low fat Greek yoghurt
- Salt & pepper to taste
- Low cal cooking spray

Method

1 Gently sauté the onion in a little low cal spray, remove from the pan and then brown off the lamb for a couple of minutes on a high heat.

2 Combine all ingredients together (except the yoghurt and spinach) in the slow cooker with the lid tightly shut and cook on low for 4-6 hours or until the lamb is tender and cooked through. 30 mins before the end of cooking add the spinach.

3 Stir through the yoghurt before serving.

CHEFS NOTE

Super-rich in iron & calcium, spinach is a super-food which is twinned beautifully in this dish with chickpeas, lemon zest and Greek inspired spices.

LAMB PILAU PAZAR

400 calories per serving

Ingredients

- 500g/1lb 2oz lean lamb cut into bite-sized chunks (any lean cut will work for this recipe)
- 1 large onion, chopped
- 1 carrot, chopped
- 1 stick celery, chopped
- 1 400g/14oz tin chopped tomatoes
- 1 tsp dried crushed chilli flakes

- 150g/5oz brown rice (use white if you prefer)
- 500ml/2 cups vegetable stock/broth
- 1 cinnamon stick or ½ teaspoon ground cinnamon
- 25g/1oz dried apricots or raisins
- Salt & pepper to taste
- Low cal cooking spray

Method

1 Gently sauté the onion in a little low cal spray, remove from the pan and then brown off the lamb for a couple of minutes on a high heat. Combine all ingredients together in the slow cooker, except the rice. Cover and cook on low for 4-6 hours, add the rice and cook for 30 mins until both the rice and lamb are tender and cooked through.

2 If any additional liquid remains, cook on a high heat with the lid off for a further 45 minutes or until the liquid is absorbed into the rice.

3 If you want to add a garnish serve with toasted pine nuts, chopped coriander/cilantro or crushed almonds.

CHEFS NOTE
Also known as pilaf, pilau is a rice-based dish now common just about everywhere. The version here has a Turkish twist to it, hence its title 'Pazar' which means 'Sunday'.

COWBOY CASSEROLE

414 calories per serving

Ingredients

- 8 lean pork sausages
- 2 400g/14oz tins mixed beans, drained
- 2 400g/14oz tins chopped tomatoes
- 1 onion, chopped
- 2 carrots, chopped
- 1 tbsp tomato puree/paste or ketchup
- 1 tsp brown sugar
- 1 tsp Dijon/mild mustard
- Low cal cooking spray

Method

1 Brown the sausages & onions in a pan with a little low cal spray. Combine all the ingredients in the slow cooker and leave to cook for 3-4 hours on high or low for 5-6 hours with the lid tightly shut. Check the sausages are properly cooked through and if you want to thicken the sauce up, leave the lid off while you cook on high for up to 45 mins.

2 Serve on its own with crusty bread or with mashed potato and green veg.

CHEFS NOTE
Loved by kids and adults alike, this is a great family meal that takes just minutes to put together.

CHILLI CON CARNE

440 calories per serving

Ingredients

- 1¼lb/550g lean mince/ground beef
- 1 400g/14oz tin chopped tomatoes
- 1 400g/14oz tin kidney beans, drained
- 1 large onion, chopped
- 250ml/1 cup beef stock/broth
- 250ml/1 cup tomato passata/sieved tomatoes
- 1 tsp each of brown sugar, oregano, cumin, chilli powder, paprika & garlic powder
- ½ tsp salt
- Low cal cooking spray

Method

1 Brown the mince and onions in a frying pan with a little low cal spray. Add all the ingredients into the slow cooker and combine well. Leave to cook on low for 5-6 hours or high for 3-4 hours with the lid tightly closed.

2 Once the meat is fully cooked through, serve with rice or tortilla chips and a dollop of low fat yoghurt or crème fraiche.

CHEFS NOTE

This is a classc dish that is perfect for the slow cooker. The kidney beans are a great source of protein and carbohydrates.

GREEN PESTO CHICKEN THIGHS

469 calories per serving

Ingredients

- 600g/1lb 2oz skinless, boneless chicken thighs
- 175g/6oz green pesto
- 250ml/1 cup buttermilk
- 1 tsp salt
- 50g/2oz asparagus spears
- 2 cloves garlic, crushed
- 1 onion, chopped

Method

1 Smother the chicken thighs in pesto and carefully combine with all the other ingredients, except the asparagus spears, in the slow cooker. Cook on low for 5-6 hours or on high for 3-4 hours with the lid tightly shut.

2 Half an hour before cooking ends add the asparagus spears. Ensure the chicken is cooked through and tender.

3 Serve with fresh green salad and crusty bread.

CHEFS NOTE

Pesto is a pounded blend of basil, cheese, pine nuts, salt and olive oil that creates a distinct taste that really complements the meaty flavour of chicken thighs. Make sure you pour any juice from the bottom of the slow cooker over the chicken before serving.

ITALIAN MEATBALLS

405
calories per
serving

Ingredients

- 650g/1lb 7oz lean minced/ground beef
- 1 slice of bread whizzed into breadcrumbs
- ½ onion, finely chopped
- Handful fresh parsley, chopped
- 1 large free range egg
- 1 clove garlic, crushed

- ½ tsp salt
- 2 400g/14oz tins chopped tomatoes
- 2 tbsp tomato puree
- 250ml/1 cup beef stock/broth
- 1 tsp each of dried basil, oregano & thyme

Method

1 Combine together the beef, breadcrumbs, egg, onion, garlic and half the salt. (You can do it with your hands or for speed put it all into a food mixer).

2 Once the ingredients are properly mixed together use your hands to shape into about 20-24 meatballs. Add all the ingredients to the slow cooker and combine well. Cover and leave to cook on low for 5-6 hours or 3-4 hours on high. Ensure the beef is well cooked and serve with spaghetti, parmesan and a green salad.

CHEFS NOTE

Meatballs are easy to make and never a disappointment to eat. The simple sauce accompanying the meat here is lovely as it is, but a dash of Worcestershire sauce or a tsp of marmite will give it additional depth.

HiiT Plan WORKOUTS

High Intensity Interval Training is a super fast and really effective way to workout. The short but intense bursts of exercise with rest in between makes your heart work harder and so increases cardio strength, improves metabolism and as a result helps your body burn more calories both during and after your workout. HiiT can also help control blood sugar levels.

It's a very efficient way to train to build a leaner, fitter body and because no equipment is required you can workout at home or just about anywhere.

We have compiled **4** core workouts to perform throughout each week. Choose one workout to perform per day and use the remaining 3 days to rest. Try to alternate between training and rest days. Each workout lasts for approximately 15 mins and a simple explanation of how to correctly perform each exercise in the set is explained in the following pages.

It's very important to warm up your muscles and joints before beginning any exercise to prevent injury and to make sure you perform each repetition to the best of your ability. Stretch for at least 2 minutes before your workout (see page 94 for stretches), then warm up by jogging on the spot for two minutes.

Always cool down and stretch again at the end of your workout.

Tips

- Warm up and cool down before and after each workout
- Have a bottle of water to drink from between sets
- Remember to breathe through each exercise
- Keep your core tight & give maximum effort
- Focus on maintaining correct posture & form for each exercise

HiiT WORKOUT ONE

- Exercise 1: **HIGH KNEES** 20 secs | 10 secs rest
- Exercise 2: **BODYWEIGHT SQUATS** 20 secs | 10 secs rest
- Exercise 3: **JUMPING JACKS** 20 secs | 10 secs rest
- Exercise 4: **SIDE LUNGE** 20 secs | 10 secs rest
- Exercise 5: **TRICEP DIPS** 20 secs | 10 secs rest
- Exercise 6: **MOUNTAIN CLIMBERS** 20 secs | 10 sec rest
- Exercise 7: **BUTT KICKS** 20 secs | 2 minute rest

Repeat for 2 more sets

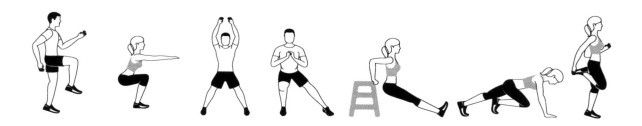

Perform each exercise as many times as possible within 20 seconds. Rest for 10 seconds then perform the next exercise again for 20 secs with a 10 sec rest in between exercises. Repeat until all 7 exercises have been completed.

Rest for 2 minutes then repeat the whole set two more times with a 2 minute rest in between.

Remember that these are high intensity workouts so try to push yourself to get as many repetitions of each exercise with the correct form within the 20 second period.

High KNEES

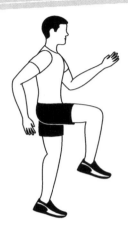 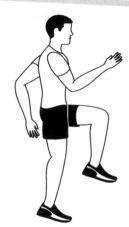

Stand straight with the feet hip width apart, looking straight ahead and arms hanging down by your side. Jump from one foot to the other at the same time lifting your knees as high as possible, hip height is advisable. The arms should be following the motion. Try holding your hands just above the hips so that your knees touch the palms of your hands as you lift your knees.

Bodyweight SQUATS

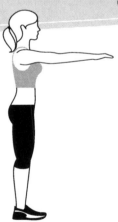 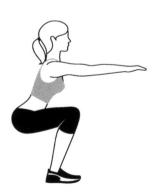

Stand with your feet shoulder width apart with your arms extended in front of you. Begin the movement by flexing your knees and hips, sitting back with your hips until your thighs are parallel with the floor in the full squat position. Quickly reverse the motion until you return to the starting position. As you keep your head and chest up.

Jumping JACKS

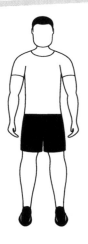
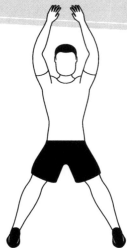

Stand with your feet together and your hands down by your side. In one motion jump your feet out to the side and raise your arms above your head. Immediately reverse by jumping back to the starting position.

Side LUNGE

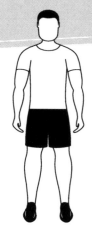
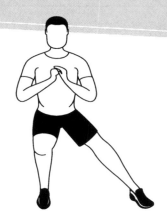

Stand with your knees and hips slightly bent, feet shoulder-width apart and the head and chest up. Keeping your left leg straight, step out to the side with your right leg and bend at your right knee transferring weight to your right side. Extend through the right leg to return to the starting position. Repeat on the left leg.

Tricep DIPS

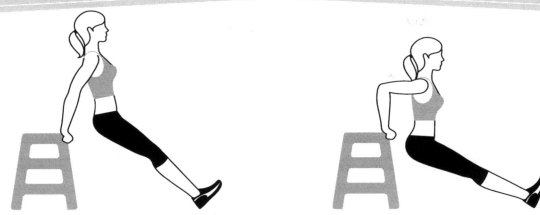

Position your hands shoulder-width apart on a secure bench or stable chair. Slide off the front of the bench with your legs extended out in front of you. Straighten your arms, keeping a slight bend in your elbows. Slowly bend your elbows to lower your body toward the floor until your elbows are at about a 90-degree angle. At this point press down into the bench or chair to straighten your elbows, returning to the starting position.

Mountain CLIMBER

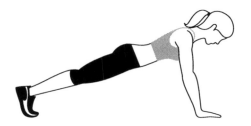 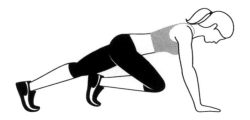

Begin in a pushup position, with your weight supported by your hands and toes. Flexing the knee and hip, bring one leg towards the corresponding arm. Explosively reverse the positions of your legs, extending the bent leg until the leg is straight and supported by the toe, and bringing the other foot up with the hip and knee flexed. Repeat in an alternating fashion.

Butt KICKS

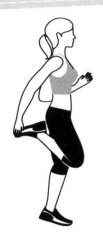 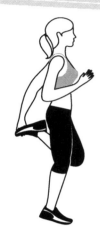

Stand with your legs shoulder-width apart and your arms bent. Flex the right knee and kick your right heel up toward your glutes. Bring the right foot back down while flexing your left knee and kicking your left foot up toward your glutes. Repeat in a continuous movement.

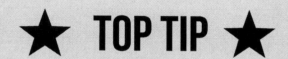

Warm up properly. By warming up your muscles you will reduce the chances of injury or strain. Warm up with jogging on the spot, gentle jumping jacks and stretches (see page 94) for at least 2 minutes.

- Exercise 1: **BURPEES** 20 secs | 10 secs rest
- Exercise 2: **JAB SQUATS** 20 secs | 10 secs rest
- Exercise 3: **MUMMY KICKS** 20 secs | 10 secs rest
- Exercise 4: **SIDE SKATER** 20 secs | 10 secs rest
- Exercise 5: **TUCK JUMP** 20 secs | 10 secs rest
- Exercise 6: **SPRINTS** 20 secs | 10 sec rest
- Exercise 7: **HEISMAN** 20 secs | 2 minute rest

Repeat for 2 more sets

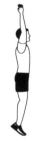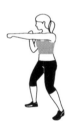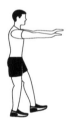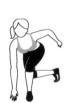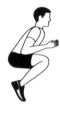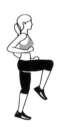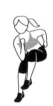

Perform each exercise as many times as possible within 20 seconds. Rest for 10 seconds then perform the next exercise again for 20 secs with a 10 sec rest in between exercises. Repeat until all 7 exercises have been completed.

Rest for 2 minutes then repeat the whole set two more times with a 2 minute rest in between.

Remember that these are high intensity workouts so try to push yourself to get as many repetitions of each exercise with the correct form within the 20 second period.

Burpees

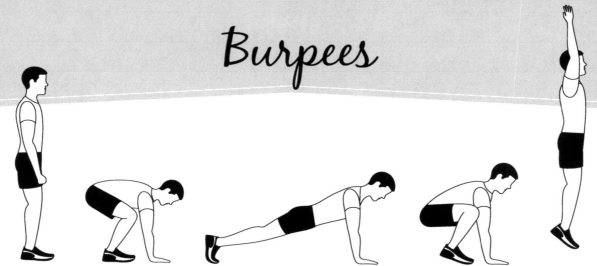

Stand with your feet shoulder-width apart, with your arms at your sides. Push your hips back, bend your knees, and lower your body into a squat before placing your hands on the floor directly in front of, and just inside, your feet. Jump your feet back to land in a plank position forming a straight line from head to toe with a straight back. Jump your feet back again so that they land just outside of your hands. Reach your arms over head and explosively jump up into the air. Land and immediately lower back into a squat for your next repetition.

Jab SQUATS

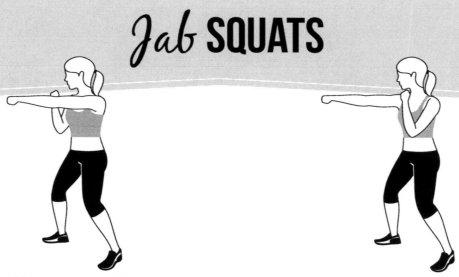

Start in a half squat position with your feet shoulder-width apart and knees slightly bent. Bring your arms up so the palms are facing the sides of your face. Clench your fists. Use sharp movements to lengthen your right arm in front in a punching motion then return to the starting position immediately punching out your left arm. Keep switching sides in a quick powerful motion.

Mummy KICKS

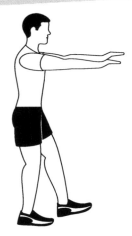 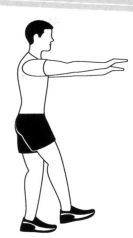

Begin by standing with your arms extended straight out in front. Perform light hop kicks with your feet while simultaneously criss-crossing your hands. Alternate the motion of your arms and hands as you swap between legs. Keep your core tight.

Side SKATER

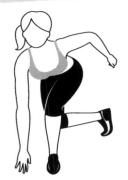 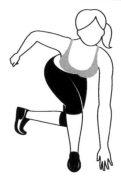

Start in a squat position with your left leg bent at the knee and your right arm parallel for balance. Your right leg is extended but still bent at the knee behind you. Jump sideways to the right, landing on your right leg. Bring your left leg behind you with your left arm extended and fingers touching the floor. Keep your back straight and your core engaged. Reverse direction by jumping to the left.

Tuck JUMP

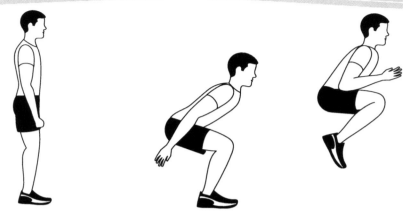

Begin in a standing position with knees slightly bent and arms at your sides. Bend your knees and lower your body quickly into a squat position, then explosively jump upwards bringing your knees up towards your chest.

Sprints

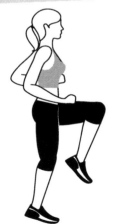 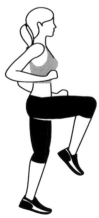

Standing with your feet shoulder-width apart, move your arms and torso as though you are running as fast as you can on the spot. Move feet and legs as little as possible avoiding twisting from side to side.

Heisman

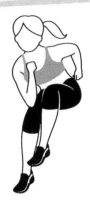 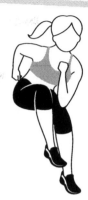

Begin by standing with feet shoulder-width apart and knees slightly bent. Jump onto your right foot while pulling your left knee up and towards the left shoulder. Next jump onto your left foot while pulling your right knee towards the right shoulder. Continue the movement in a quick motion, switching between legs.

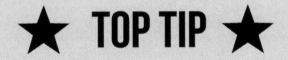

★ TOP TIP ★

Use a timer or stopwatch to precisely time each exercise and your rest time. There are many free apps available online. Try searching for 'tabata timer app'.

HiiT WORKOUT THREE

- Exercise 1: **SIT UPS** 20 secs | 10 secs rest
- Exercise 2: **BICYCLE CRUNCH** 20 secs | 10 secs rest
- Exercise 3: **MUMMY KICKS** 20 secs | 10 secs rest
- Exercise 4: **JAB SQUATS** 20 secs | 10 secs rest
- Exercise 5: **LATERALS** 20 secs | 10 secs rest
- Exercise 6: **MOUNTAIN CLIMBER** 20 secs | 10 sec rest
- Exercise 7: **TAP UP** 20 secs | 2 minute rest

Repeat for 2 more sets

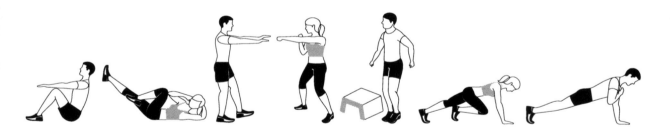

Perform each exercise as many times as possible within 20 seconds. Rest for 10 seconds then perform the next exercise again for 20 secs with a 10 sec rest in between exercises. Repeat until all 7 exercises have been completed.

Rest for 2 minutes then repeat the whole set two more times with a 2 minute rest in between.

Remember that these are high intensity workouts so try to push yourself to get as many repetitions of each exercise with the correct form within the 20 second period.

Sit UPS

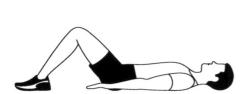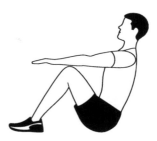

Lie on your back with your knees bent and your arms extended at your sides. and your feet flat on the floor. Engage your core and slowly curl your upper back off the floor towards your knees with your arms extended out. Roll back down to the starting position.

Bicycle CRUNCH

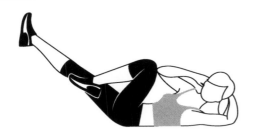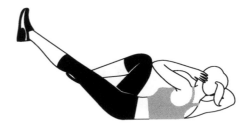

Lie face up and place your hands at the side of your head (do not pull on the back of your head). Make sure your core is tight and the small of your back is pushed hard against the floor. Lift your knees in toward your chest while lifting your shoulder blades off the floor. Rotate to the right, bringing the left elbow towards the right knee as you extend the other leg into the air. Switch sides, bringing the right elbow towards the left knee. Alternate each side in a pedaling motion..

Mummy KICKS

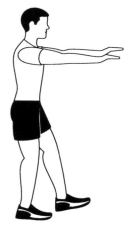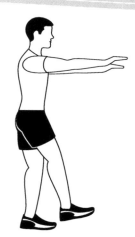

Begin by standing with your arms extended straight out in front. Perform light hop kicks with your feet while simultaneously criss-crossing your hands. Alternate the motion of your arms and hands as you swap between legs. Keep your core tight.

Jab SQUATS

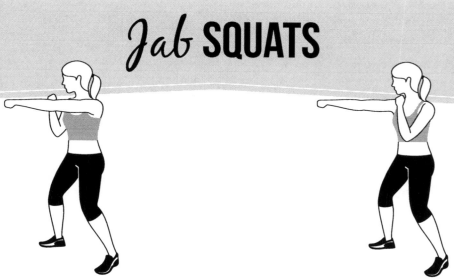

Start in a half squat position with your feet shoulder-width apart and knees slightly bent. Bring your arms up so the palms are facing the sides of your face. Clench your fists. Use sharp movements to lengthen your right arm in front in a punching motion then return to the starting position immediately punching out your left arm. Keep switching sides in a quick powerful motion.

Laterals

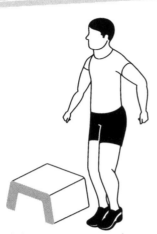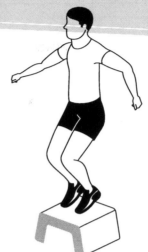

Stand beside a step or box. Position into a quarter squat then jump up and over to the right landing on the box with both feet landing together. Bring your knees high enough to ensure your feet clear the box. Jump over to the other side and repeat, this time jumping to the left.

Mountain CLIMBER

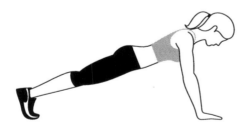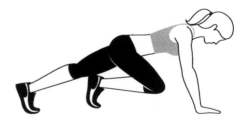

Begin in a pushup position, with your weight supported by your hands and toes. Flexing the knee and hip, bring one leg towards the corresponding arm. Explosively reverse the positions of your legs, extending the bent leg until the leg is straight and supported by the toe, and bringing the other foot up with the hip and knee flexed. Repeat in an alternating fashion.

Tap UPS

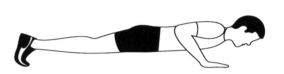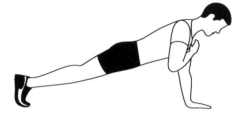

Begin in a pushup/plank position with your hands slightly wider than shoulder-width apart. Bend your elbows to lower your body to the floor just like a normal pushup. Pause, press back up to the starting position then tap one shoulder with the opposite side's hand. Repeat tapping the opposite shoulder.

★ **TOP TIP** ★

Work as hard as you can in each 20 sec burst. This is high intensity training so give maximum effort while maintaining correct form for each exercise.

HiiT WORKOUT FOUR

- Exercise 1: **PRESS UPS** 20 secs | 10 secs rest
- Exercise 2: **SQUAT LUNGE** 20 secs | 10 secs rest
- Exercise 3: **STANDING STRAIGHT LEG BICYCLE** 20 secs | 10 secs rest
- Exercise 4: **TUCK JUMPS** 20 secs | 10 secs rest
- Exercise 5: **STANDING MOUNTAIN CLIMBERS** 20 secs | 10 secs rest
- Exercise 6: **BURPEES** 20 secs | 10 sec rest
- Exercise 7: **SCISSOR JUMPS** 20 secs | 2 minute rest

Repeat for 2 more sets

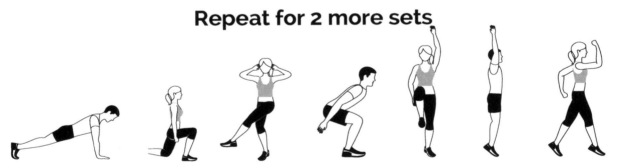

Perform each exercise as many times as possible within 20 seconds or hold for the desired length of time depending on the drill. Rest for 10 seconds then perform the next exercise again for 20 secs with a 10 sec rest in between exercises. Repeat until all 7 exercises have been completed.

Rest for 2 minutes then repeat the whole set two more times with a 2 minute rest in between.

Press UPS

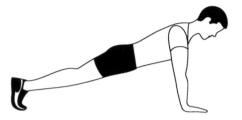

Begin in a high plank position with your hands shoulder-width apart. Lower your body ensuring you keep it aligned and look ahead to avoid strain in the neck. When your chest brushes the floor push back up. If you find this move difficult, start with your knees on the floor lowering only your upper torso.

Squat LUNGE

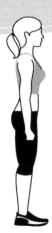
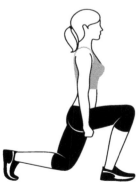

Stand upright with feet hip-width apart and arms at your sides. Take a controlled step forward with your right leg, keeping balance so that both knees are at 90 degree angles. Make sure your hips are low and back is straight. Push back with your right leg to the starting position. Repeat on left leg.

Standing Straight Leg BICYCLE

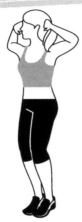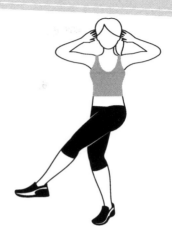

Begin by standing tall, hands touching the sides of your head but not clasped, feet shoulder-width apart. Opening your elbows wide, bring your right elbow down while simultaneously raising your left knee till they meet. Return to the starting position then repeat with left elbow to right knee. Opposite elbows go to opposite knees.

Tuck JUMP

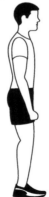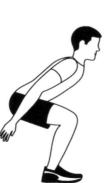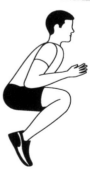

Begin in a standing position with knees slightly bent and arms at your sides. Bend your knees and lower your body quickly into a squat position, then explosively jump upwards bringing your knees up towards your chest.

Standing MOUNTAIN CLIMBER

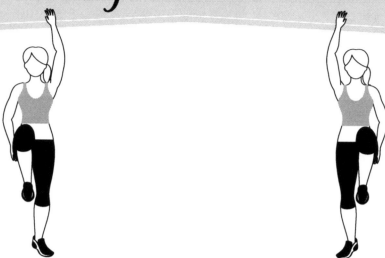

Begin by standing with feet shoulder-width apart and arms by your side. Bring your left knee up to waist level while extending your right arm to the sky. Return to the starting position then repeat this time raising your right knee and left arm. Keep alternating sides in a climbing motion.

Burpees

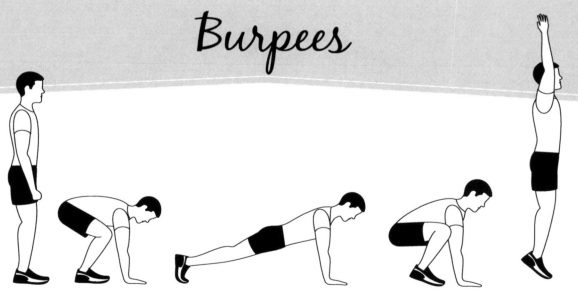

Lie on your back and extend your arms out to the side. Raise your knees and feet so they create a 90-degree angle. Contract your abdominals and exhale as you lift your hips off the floor. Your knees will move toward your head. Try to keep your knees at a right angle. Inhale and slowly lower.

Scissor JUMPS

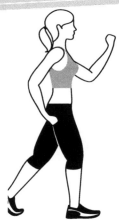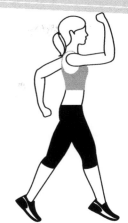

Begin by standing with right foot approx. 2 feet in front of left. Right arm should be extended behind you and left arm in front of you with elbows bent as if in a running position. Quickly jump up while switching arm and leg positions while in the air, landing with left foot in front of right foot and right arm in front of your body, left arm behind you. Continue alternating arms and legs while jumping.

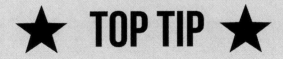

★ TOP TIP ★

Keep your core tight! By keeping your abdominal area firm, not only are you working the ab muscles but also keeping a strong mid-section which is vital for balance and control.

Straight Leg Calf STRETCH

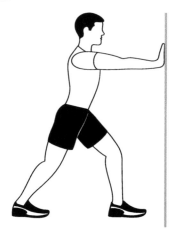 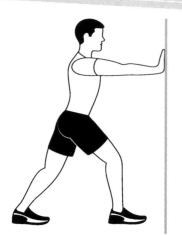

Place both hands on a wall with arms extended. Lean against the wall with right leg bent forward and left leg extended behind with knee straight and feet positioned directly forward. Push rear heal to floor and move hips slightly forward holding the stretch for 10 secs. Repeat with opposite leg.

Shoulder STRETCH

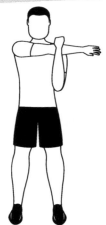 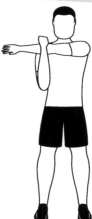

The right arm is placed over the left shoulder. Position the wrist on your left arm to the elbow of your right arm gently pushing towards the shoulder. Swap shoulders.

Standing Quadricep STRETCH

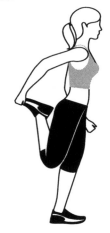 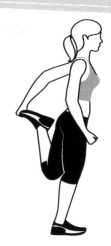

Begin by standing with your feet hip-width apart. Bend your right leg backwards grasping the right foot to bring your heel toward your buttocks. Hold for 5-10 secs then repeat for left leg. Use your opposite arm to balance if need be.

Lower Back STRETCH

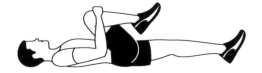 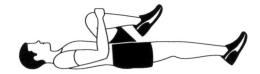

Begin by lying flat on your back with toes pointed upward. Slowly bend your right knee and pull your leg up to you chest, wrapping your arms around your thigh and hands clasped around the knee or shin. Gently pull the knee towards your chest and hold for 10 secs. Repeat on left leg.

Cat Cow STRETCH

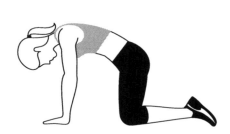 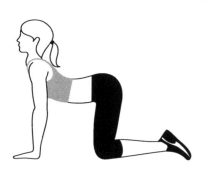

Begin with your hands and knees on the floor. Exhale while rounding your spine up towards the ceiling, pulling your belly button up towards your spine, and engaging your core. Inhale while arching your back and letting your tummy relax.

· 🍎 **CookNation** ·

Other
COOKNATION
TITLES

If you enjoyed **The** *Skinny* **Slow Cooker/Fast Fitness Recipe & Workout Book** you may also be interested in other *Skinny* titles in the CookNation series.

Visit **www.bellmackenzie.com** to browse the full catalogue.

19594275R00056

Printed in Poland
by Amazon Fulfillment
Poland Sp. z o.o., Wrocław